Musculoskeletal and Sports Physiotherapy Practical Record Book For Bachelor of Physiotherapy

Dr. Smruti Swagatika Dash, PT
MPT (Musculoskeletal & Sports Physiotherapy)
MIAP, M-MTFI
Assistant Professor
Narayana Hrudayalaya Institute of Physiotherapy
Hosur Road
Bangalore - 560099

PEEPEE
PUBLISHERS AND DISTRIBUTORS (P) LTD.

Published by:
Pawaninder P. Vij
Peepee Publishers and Distributors (P) Ltd.
Head Office: 160, Shakti Vihar, Pitam Pura
New Delhi-110 034

Correspondence Address:

7/31, Ansari Road, Daryaganj
New Delhi-110002 (India)

Ph: 65195868, 41512412, 9811156083

e-mail: **peepee160@yahoo.co.in**

e-mail: **peepee160@gmail.com**

www.peepeepub.com

First Edition: 2018

ISBN: 978-81-8445-235-8

Preface

This book was created to aid the undergraduate physiotherapy students to have a concise Practical manual. It will guide them in clinical scenario in taking down the assessments. They would also know the differential diagnosis of common conditions.

My dear physiotherapy students can document all clinically relevant parameters in the record book, which they can preserve for their future reference. It would be definitely helpful for their undergraduate practical examination.

It is specially designed to make orthopaedics physiotherapy practical more lively.

Dr. Smruti Swagatika Dash, PT

Acknowledgements

I would like to thank Almighty God for giving me strength in accomplishing this work.

I owe my deepest gratitude to my parents (Dr. Gyanendranath Dash and Prof. Mrs. Smiti Sudha Tripathy), my husband Mr. Ansuman Rath (Marketing Consultant), my in-laws Dr. Debi Prasana Rath, Mrs Snigdha Rath and my brother Suswagat Dash.

Loads of love to my little champ, my son Aayansh Rath for instilling me with all positive energy.

I would like to thank my family for their constant motivation. Thanks to Dr. (Mrs.) S.N Tripathy, Dr. Eteesradha Tripathy, Mr. Satyendranath Dash, Mrs. Jyotsna Rani Dash and Mr. Srikrishna Tripathy for being with me in all my good and bad times.

I would like to express my sincere thanks to Peepee Publishers for publishing my work. My humble obligation to my teachers and my patients who taught me each and every aspect of physiotherapy.

Dr. Smruti Swagatika Dash, PT

Musculoskeletal and Sports Physiotherapy
Practical Record Book For
Bachelor of Physiotherapy
Third Year

STUDENT NAME:

UNIVERSITY REGISTRATION NUMBER:

STATUS:
REMARKS:

MUSCULOSKELETAL AND SPORTS PHYSIOTHERAPY HOD

....

PRINCIPAL

....

Contents

PRACTICAL 1: SOAP Assessment

PRACTICAL 2: Physiotherapy Assessment of Orthopaedic conditions

PRACTICAL 3: BASCIC ORTHOPEDICS:

1) DRAW A BONE & LABEL ITS PARTS:

2) ROM OF ALL JOINTS:

3) END FEEL:

4) CAPSULAR PATTERNS FOR ALL THE JOINTS:

PRACTICAL 4:

1) Assessment of Fractures:

2) Fracture healing:

3) Fracture complications – General & PT management:

4) Fracture immobilisers:

5) Internal & external fixators:

PRACTICAL 5:

1) Assessment of cervical spine:

2) Differential diagnosis for cervical Pain.

3) PT management for cervical pain syndrome.

4) Special tests for the cervical vertebra.

PRACTICAL 6:

1) Assessment of lumbar spine.

2) Differential diagnosis of lumbar spine.

3) PT management for low back pain.

4) Special tests for lumbar spine.

PRACTICAL 7:

1) Assessment of shoulder pain.

2) Differential diagnosis for shoulder pain.

3) PT management for:

a) Frozen shoulder

b) Rotator cuff tear

c) **Supraspinatus tendinitis**

d) Shoulder dislocation & recurrent shoulder dislocation

PRACTICAL 8: ELBOW COMPLEX

1) Assessment of elbow pain.

2) Differential diagnosis for elbow pain.

3) Special tests for elbow region.

4) PT management for tennis elbow.

PRACTICAL 9: WRIST & HAND

1) Assessment of wrist pain.

2) Differential diagnosis for wrist pain

3) Special test for wrist & hand.

4) PT management for wrist sprain.

5) PT management for flexor tendon injuries.

6) PT management for extension tendon injuries.

PRACTICAL 10: HIP COMPLEX

1) Assessment for hip pain.

2) **Differential diagnosis for hip pain (ant, post & lat).**

3) Special tests for hip region.

4) PT management for hip dislocation.

5) PT management for THR (Hip arthroplasty)

6) PT management for hip OA.

7) PT management for piriformis syndrome.

PRACTICAL 11: KNEE COMPLEX

1) Assessment for knee pain.

2) Differential diagnosis for knee pain (ant, post, lat)

3) Special tests for knee pain.

4) PT management for knee OA.

5) PT management for TKR (Knee arthroplasty).

6) PT management for meniscal injury.

7) PT management for ACL injury.

8) PT management for PCL injury.

9) PT management for MCL injury.

10) PT management for LCL injury.

11) PT management for patellar tendon ruptures.

12) Patellectomy rehabilitation.

PRACTICAL 12: ANKLE & FOOT

1) Assessment for ankle pain.

2) Differential diagnosis for ankle pain.

3) Special tests for ankle pain.

4) PT management for ankle sprain.

5) PT management for TA rupture.

PRACTICAL 13: POSTURE.

1) Assessment of posture.

2) Common postural deviations in sagittal plane & frontal plane.

3) PT management for forward head posture.

PRACTICAL 14: GAIT.

1) Assessment of Gait.

2) Determinants of gait.

3) Common pathological gaits.

4) Gait deviations with prosthesis.

PRACTICAL 15: AMPUTATION, PROSTHESIS & ORTHOSIS

1) Amputation- levels, indications & contraindications.

2) Stump care.

3) Complications of amputation & its management.

4) Preprosthetic training.

5) Prosthetic care & fit.

6) Types & parts of prosthesis.

7) Orthosis – indications.

8) Orthotic shoe.

9) Types of spinal orthosis.

10) Types of upper limb orthosis.

11) Types of lower limb orthosis.

PRACTICAL 16: CEREBRAL PALSY.

1) Milestones of development.

2) Neonatal primitive reflexes.

3) Assessment of CP.

4) Common deformities in CP, its surgery & PT management.

PRACTICAL 17: NEUROMUSCULAR DISORDERS:

1) Assessment and management of poliomyelitis.

2) **Assessment and management of spinal dysraphism.**

3) Assessment and management of leprosy.

PRACTICAL 18: INFLAMMATORY & DEGENERATIVE CONDITION:

1) PT assessment & management for OA.

2) PT assessment & management for RA.

3) PT assessment & management for AS.

4) PT assessment & management for perthes disease.

5) PT assessment & management for gout.

6) Differentiate between OA, RA & AS.

PRACTICAL 19: MANUAL THERAPY

1) Maitland school of thought.

2) McKenzie school of thought.

PRACTICAL 20: LOW BACK PAIN & NECK PAIN

1) PT management for Low Back Pain.

2) Differential diagnosis for LBP.

3) Ergonomic advice for Low back pain.

4) PT management for neck pain.

5) Ergonomic advice for neck pain.

6) PT management for spondylolisthesis.

PRACTICAL 21: SPECIAL FRACTURES & MISCELLANEOUS

1) PT assessment & management for SUPRACONDYLAR # OF HUMERUS.

2) PT assessment & management for COLLE'S #.

3) PT assessment & management for SMITH'S #.

4) PT assessment & management for SCAPHOID #.

5) PT assessment & management for # NECK OF FEMUR.

6) PT assessment & management for # OF TROCHANTERS.

7) PT assessment & management for # SHAFT OF FEMUR.

8) PT assessment & management for POTT'S #.

9) PT assessment & management for CERVICAL SPINE #.

10) PT assessment & management for THORACIS SPINE #.

11) PT assessment & management for LUMBAR SPINE #.

12) PT assessment & management for POTT'S SPINE.

13) Contusions.

14) Burn injuries of hand.

15) Recurrent dislocation of patella.

16) PT Management for Frozen shoulder.

17) PT management for carpal tunnel syndrome.

18) PT management of plantar fasciitis.

NOTES:

NOTES:

NOTES: